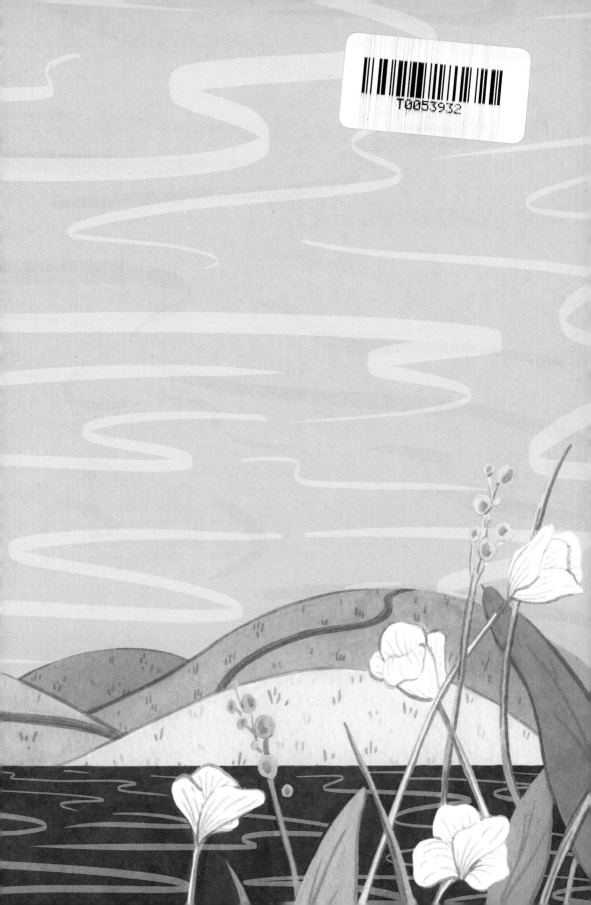

To Wolf, Hector, Orson, Gerry and Jo. Thank you.
- Alice

To Paul, Julia, Roger, Harry, Toby and Alice
- Christy

To Ashley
- Eleanor

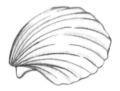

The Sleepy Pebble and Other Stories © Flying Eye Books 2019.

First edition published in 2019 by Flying Eye Books, an imprint of Nobrow Ltd.
27 Westgate Street, London E8 3RL.

Text © Professor Alice Gregory and Christy Kirkpatrick 2019
Illustrations © Eleanor Hardiman 2019

Book design by Bia Melo

Professor Alice Gregory and Christy Kirkpatrick have asserted their rights under the Copyright,
Designs and Patents Act, 1988, to be identified as the Authors of this Work.

Published in the US by Nobrow (US) Inc.

Printed in Latvia on FSC® certified paper.

1 3 5 7 9 10 8 6 4 2

ISBN: 978-1-911171-8-12

www.flyingeyebooks.com

THE SLEEPY PEBBLE

AND OTHER STORIES

CALMING TALES TO READ AT BEDTIME

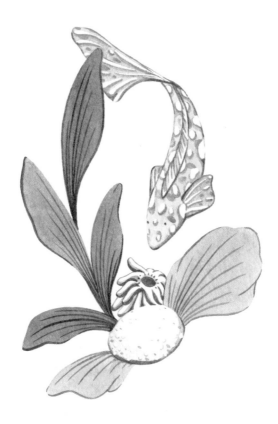

Written by Professor Alice Gregory and Christy Kirkpatrick
Illustrated by Eleanor Hardiman

FLYING EYE BOOKS

London | New York

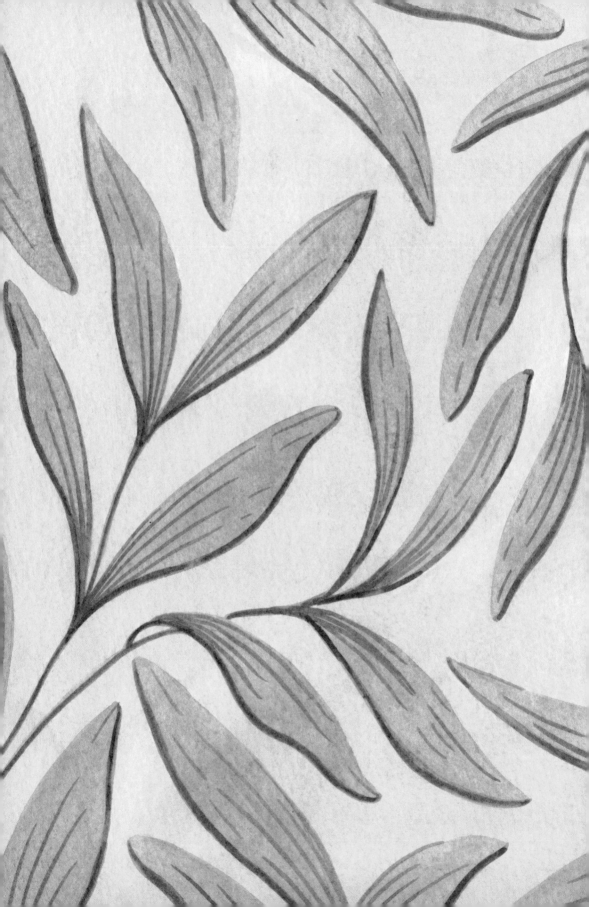

CONTENTS

AN INTRODUCTION FOR GROWN-UPS

Many families have a bedtime routine, probably involving a bath and stories. Then, us adults turn off the light and expect our children to go to sleep. The last part of bedtime – when we expect children to be quiet and fall asleep – can be a time when things go wrong. Our children might tell us they don't want to go to sleep. They might ask for more stories or keep chatting about whatever is on their mind. It's easy for us to become exasperated. How can our children possibly not be sleepy when they have had such a busy day, it's already well past their bedtime and we are exhausted ourselves?

One possibility is that our children might be tired, but in a state of 'arousal', meaning a physical and mental state of being alert and reactive to stimuli. They might have just read the most exciting story about a roller coaster ride and are imagining themselves whizzing round at high speed. They might remember having been tickled earlier in the day and are still laughing at the feeling. No wonder our children can't sleep: high levels of arousal are incompatible with sleep. But, with a bit of help, they can unwind so that they are in a state that is better suited to falling asleep.

What might help?

The Sleepy Pebble and Other Stories is designed to help children relax before bedtime. Useful techniques are embedded in calm and peaceful stories. Each story contains three elements: imagery, muscle relaxation and mindfulness.

Imagery

Imagery encourages children to create a place in their minds. In order to seem realistic, children are encouraged to consider a scene in plenty of detail. They might think about the sounds and smells they encounter. Research in adults with insomnia has found that those asked to imagine a scene in a great amount of detail fell asleep more quickly than those given no instructions. Imagery is also sometimes used in schools to help children relax. This technique may be useful because keeping an image in the mind uses up 'cognitive space', which can therefore not be filled with thoughts that may keep children awake.

Muscle Relaxation

Progressive muscle relaxation is a technique whereby different groups of muscles are tensed and then released. Doing so can help children to notice how different it feels when they are tense, compared to when they are relaxed. A review of non-pharmacological treatments for adults with chronic insomnia from the American Academy of Sleep Medicine, concluded that progressive muscle relaxation is a method that works. This technique has also been used with children. We have developed a brief version of this established technique to use in the context of the stories.

Mindfulness

Mindfulness refers to 'being in the moment' without judgement. This means noticing three things: how our bodies feel, the thoughts that are passing through our minds and the environment around us – like feeling the temperature of the air or noticing nearby sounds. However, mindfulness is about more than just paying attention to the present moment: *how* we pay attention is important. Mindfulness involves awareness of what is currently being experienced with openness, curiosity, self-compassion and non-judgement. Paying attention with the wrong attitude – for example, by being critical or anxious about what is happening – is not helpful. Increased levels of mindfulness have been associated with better sleep quality in both adults and children, and mindfulness-based therapy is often used as a component of therapies designed to improve sleep in adults (such as Cognitive Behavioural Therapy for Insomnia). It is also sometimes used in school settings to increase well-being. Mindfulness could help children to sleep for multiple reasons, for example its ability to reduce anxiety and relax the body – which could have a knock-on positive effect on sleep.

WILL THIS BOOK HELP?

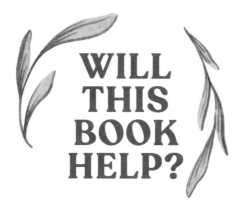

When developing this book over a few years, we drew upon scientific literature. We also contacted other sleep experts, psychologists, mindfulness experts, parents and children themselves about our ideas and have shared early draft sections of this book widely, receiving plenty of feedback. We also conducted a small pilot study where we invited 100 families (who had at least one child aged between 3 and 11 years of age) to take part. We asked the families to read a story (an earlier draft of *The Sleepy Pebble*) for three consecutive nights. At the end of those nights, we asked the families to answer a questionnaire providing feedback about many aspects of the story, such as its length and whether they thought it should be illustrated. Seventy adults participating in the study responded. We asked many questions, but for one key question: "Overall, what effect do you think the story had on your child/children's sleep?", parents responded that for 80 of the 104 (77%) children taking part the story had a 'very positive' or 'slightly positive' effect*. They also flagged areas that could be improved (such as adding illustrations and information for adults reading the story). The book has been adapted based on the feedback. Positive feedback does not mean that this book will work for all children. Every child is unique – and what is helpful for one child may not be helpful for another. We would recommend adding this to your bedtime routine if you and your children find it useful and encourage you only to use sections of the book that you consider to be appropriate for your children. For children with physical or mental health difficulties, a healthcare provider should be consulted before using any techniques included in this book.

---

*Parents also reported that for 21/104 (20%) the book seemed to have no effect; for 3/104 (3%) the book seemed to have a slightly negative/extremely negative effect/did not comment. Our study had limitations (e.g. there was no control group, and we used subjective retrospective reports. Recruitment was also conducted via social media meaning that the authors were known to some of the participants). Nonetheless, the overall results were promising.

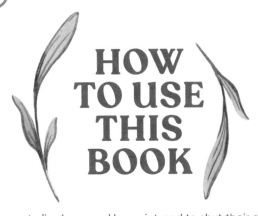

HOW TO USE THIS BOOK

You might want to consider the tips at the end of this book to help you create an appropriate environment before you start reading one of our stories. We recommend that you choose one each night and read it to your child as the last story before bedtime. When it is time to start reading the story, ask your child to lie down and be quiet and to shut their eyes, if they are happy to do so. Try to make your voice calm and soothing, and read the stories slowly and quietly. Novelty can be arousing, so when you present a story to your child for the first time, it may not have the desired effect. Your child might be excited by the new book and want to interact with it. Please do not worry about this. When you first read the book, encourage your child to look at it and answer any questions that they have – explain to them that this is a different type of book to those that you usually read and that over time you would like them to be quiet and peaceful when listening to their 'sleepy book'. Hopefully after the novelty has worn off, the stories will help your child relax before falling asleep. You may find it useful to read the Questions and Answers listed on page 79 for further advice when using this book. Once the story is finished, keep the lights dim and the bedroom calm and quiet. Now is the time to say goodnight and leave the room so that you can let your child go to sleep. We wish you a peaceful night.

Professor Alice Gregory
Christy Kirkpatrick

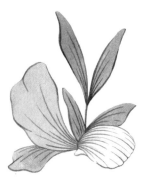

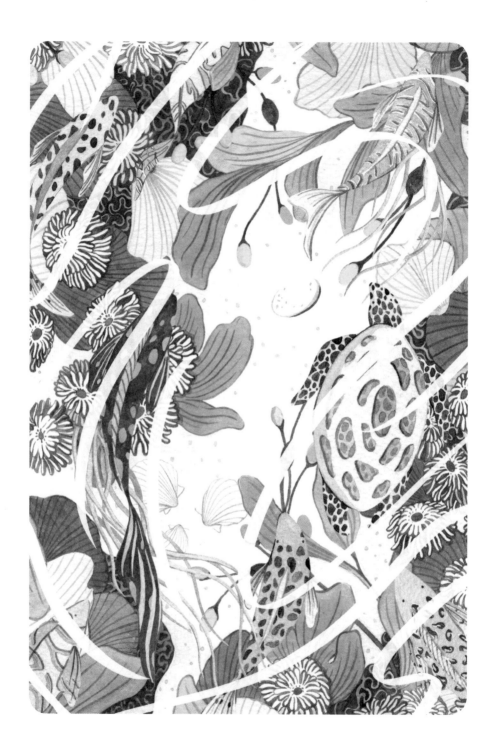

THE SLEEPY PEBBLE

Pebble wakes, as he does every morning, safe and snug in his sea bed. He opens one eye, then he opens the other. He yawns and stretches, and stretches and yawns. He sleepily rubs his eyes and enjoys feeling warm and cosy. He thinks about the day ahead.

Let's think about little Pebble.

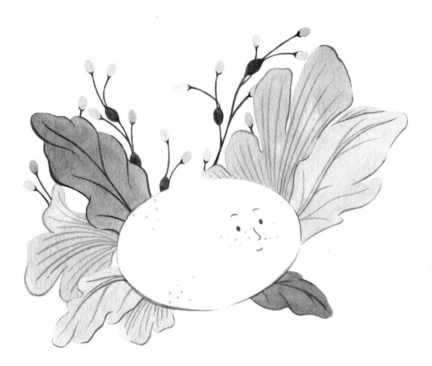

IMAGERY

Be as quiet as you can and think about Pebble in his sea bed. Try to picture him yawning and stretching, stretching and yawning.

Think about Pebble's sea bed. Be still and calm and think about the ocean floor on which he is lying. Imagine a blanket or some thick seaweed keeping Pebble warm.

Staying quiet, look out beyond Pebble's sea bed and into the clear water. Imagine the waves rolling out to sea. Listen to the sounds the waves make.

Listen really hard.

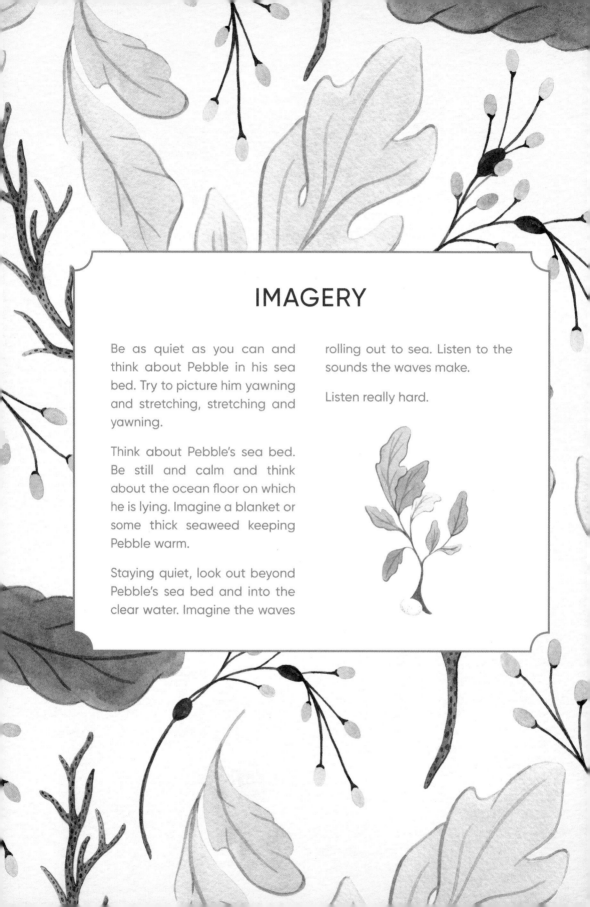

Pebble usually spends the morning playing with his brothers and sisters, but today he feels like a change.

He eats breakfast, brushes his teeth and shuffles outside.

"Do you want to join us, Pebble?" his brothers and sisters ask. "We are playing hide-and-seek. We are hiding and peeping, peeping and hiding."

Pebble loves hide-and-seek. Usually he would join in, but today he wants to do something different.

"Thanks, but no thanks," he says. "I feel like a bit of a change." Pebble nods goodbye and continues on his way.

After a while, Pebble spots his friends, dancing and shuffling, shuffling and dancing.

"Do you want to join us, Pebble?" his friends ask, calling him over. "We are practising our dance steps for the Grand Pebble Ball."

Pebble loves dancing. Usually he would join in, but not today.

"No, thank you," he says. "I'm off on an adventure."

Pebble nods goodbye and continues on his way.

After a while, Pebble sees a school of fish swimming past silently.

"Do you want to come with us?" the fish ask him. "We're off to explore the sea. We are splashing and diving, diving and splashing." Pebble smiles.

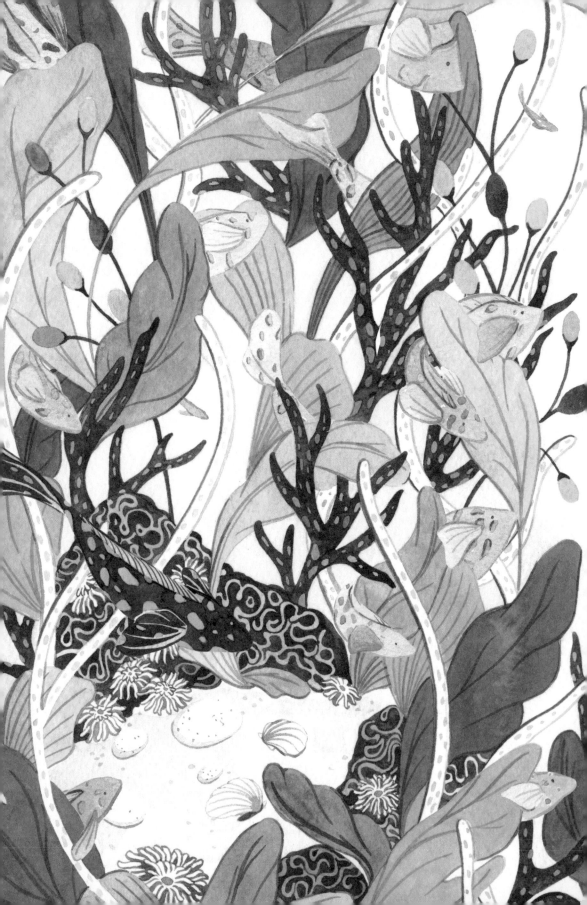

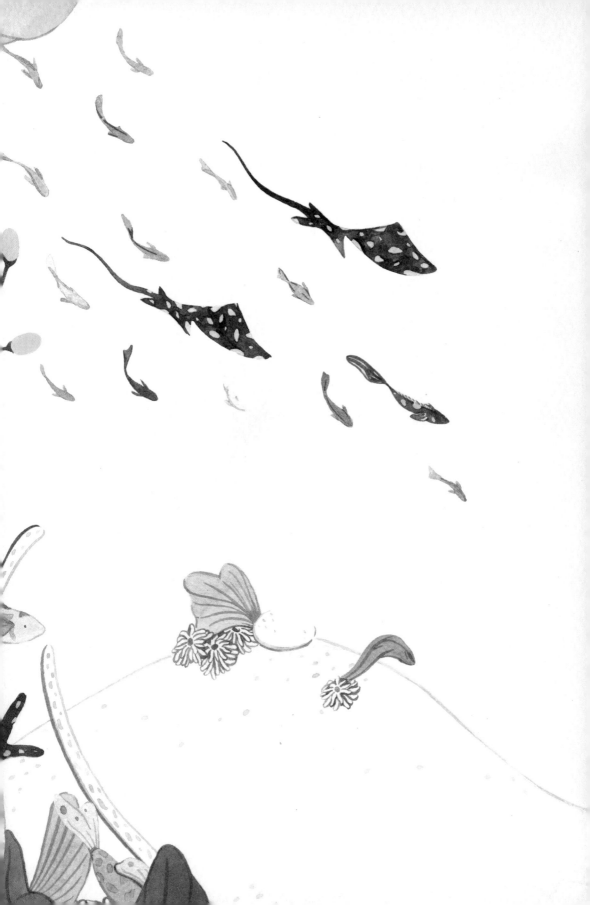

"I want to do something different," he thinks, "and this is something different."

"Yes, please," he says, and a golden fish lets Pebble climb on to her back.

Pebble loves swimming with the fish. He sees fish that are big and small, red and green and silver and gold. He hears the quiet chatter of sea creatures and enjoys the feeling of the cool sea against him.

"This is great fun," Pebble says, and his new friends agree. They have a wonderful day together exploring the ocean and all the things it has to offer.

The youngest fish start to yawn. It is time to start getting ready to go home.

"Where is your home, Pebble?" the fish asks. "I can take you there."

Pebble is starting to feel tired. He wants to go home.

Let's help Pebble get to his sea bed at the bottom of the ocean.

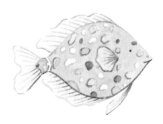

MUSCLE RELAXATION

Imagine that you have Pebble in your hand and that every time you squeeze him, it pushes him towards his home.

For this to work, it is really important that you are very quiet. Be quiet and lie very still. Be as calm and as quiet and as still as you can be.

Now listen. Imagine you have Pebble in the palm of your hand. Squeeze Pebble as hard as you can. That's right, keep squeezing. Now relax your hand.

Take a really big breath in through your nose and slowly let it out. Take a deep breath in ... and a slow breath out... Relax for five, four, three, two, one. Feel how sleepy your hand is now.

Now imagine Pebble is in your other hand. Remember to be as quiet as you can for the squeezing to work. Squeeze Pebble as hard as you can. That's right, keep squeezing. Now relax your hand. Take a deep breath in ... and a slow breath out... Relax for five, four, three, two, one. Feel how sleepy your hand is now.

Now imagine Pebble is under your foot, right under your toes. Squeeze your foot. That's right, keep squeezing. Now relax your foot.

Take a deep breath in ... and a slow breath out... Relax for five, four, three, two, one. Feel how sleepy your foot is now.

Now for the other foot. Squeeze your foot. That's right, keep squeezing. Now relax your foot. Take a deep breath in ... and a slow breath out... Relax for five, four, three, two, one. Feel how sleepy your foot is now.

Finally, imagine that you *are* little pebble and squeeze your whole body. Keep squeezing and then relax your whole body.

Take a deep breath in ... and a slow breath out... Relax for five, four, three, two, one. Feel how relaxed your whole body is now.

Well done. Pebble is home safely. He is feeling very tired now.

Pebble has something to eat, then brushes his teeth. He goes to his sea bed and gets in. He is safe, snug and relaxed.

Pebble yawns and stretches and stretches and yawns. He closes one eye and then the other. He enjoys feeling warm and still. He thinks about the day he has spent swimming with the fish. Then his mum and dad come to read him a story and say goodnight.

"Did you enjoy doing something different?" Mum asks him.

"I did," Pebble says. "It's good to try new things, sometimes."

"That's true," Mum agrees. "You did a great job of being brave and trying something new."

Pebble pulls his blanket up to his chin and feels very pleased to be safe and snug in his sea bed.

"I like doing things that are different," Pebble says, "but sometimes, and especially when I'm going to sleep, I like doing things that *aren't* different."

"Me too," Dad says gently.

"At bedtime," Pebble says thoughtfully, "I like doing things that are just the same." Mum agrees. She kisses Pebble goodnight and leaves the room, so that Pebble can fall asleep, as he falls asleep every evening, safe and snug in his sea bed.

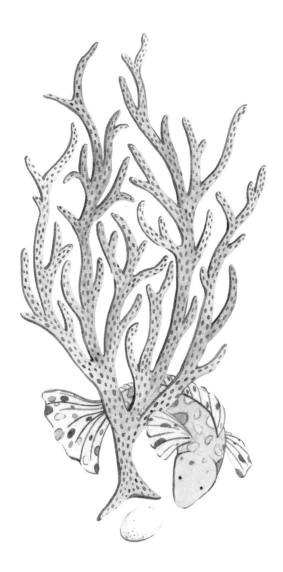

MINDFULNESS

Now it's time for *you* to close *your* eyes. For the next few minutes, you are going to relax and get all cosy and snug, just like Pebble in his sea bed.

Try and get comfortable.

Choose a position that makes you feel relaxed. You could lie on your side or on your back. That's right, get really comfortable in your bed and relax.

Let your head rest on your pillow. Think really carefully about how your pillow feels under your head. Don't speak, but take a few moments to notice what is happening right here, right now. There is no right or wrong way to feel.

Staying quiet, think to yourself whether you feel hot or cold.

Let's think about your breathing now. You might feel air coming in through your nose when you breathe, or you may feel your tummy filling up like a balloon and then deflating.

Take a deep breath in.
Now slowly let it out.
Take a deep breath in.
Now let it out.

Take a deep breath in …
and a slow breath out.
In … and out…

Staying still, notice how your arms feel. They might feel tired or they might feel relaxed. There is no right or wrong way to feel.

Without moving, think really carefully about how your legs feel. They might feel tired from running and moving all day, or they might feel rested.

Think about what is happening right here, right now. Feel the air coming into your tummy, and going out again.

Take a deep breath in …
and a slow breath out.
In … and out…

Let yourself sleep whenever you are ready.

Goodnight, Sleepy Pebble.

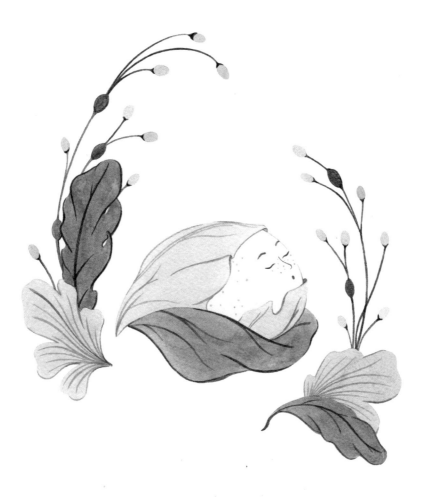

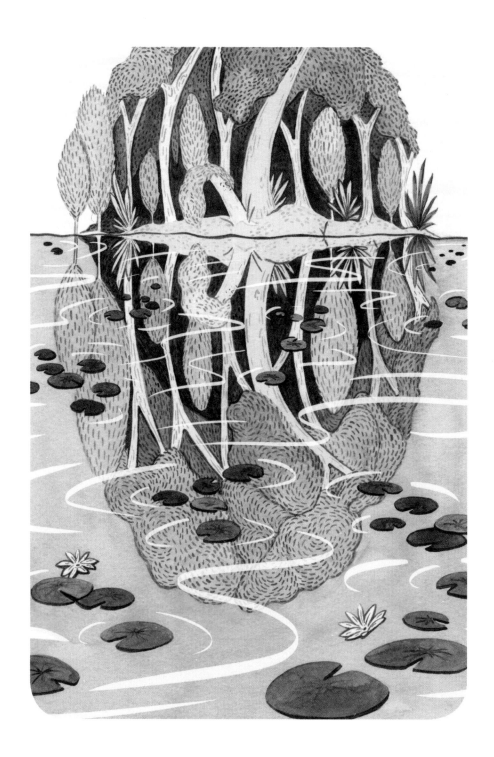

THE TREE WHO WANTED TO STAY UP LATE

Willow was a small but strong tree, with light green curls that poured over a shiny, shimmering lake at the edge of a forest. She had been friends with Wise Old Tree, who was as tall as she was small, for as long as she could remember. However, there was one thing about Wise Old Tree that Willow could never understand.

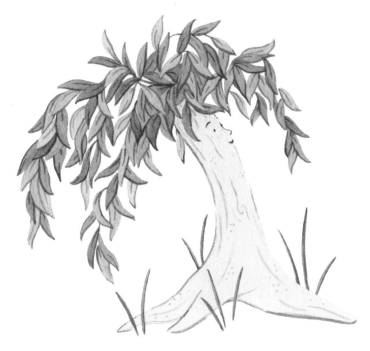

"Why do you always go to sleep so early?" Willow asked Wise Old Tree every evening, as he got himself ready for bed. "When I'm grown up, I want to stay up late and see what happens at night-time in the forest."

"Night-time is for night creatures, like owls and bats," Wise Old Tree told Willow each time she asked. "Us trees need our sleep. We need to keep our branches strong, so that the birds can build their nests here. We need to keep our roots strong, so that we do not tumble into the lake. And we need to grow lots of leaves, to provide shelter for all our animal friends who live in the forest." Let's think about Willow and Wise Old Tree in the forest.

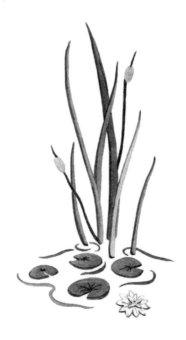

IMAGERY

Be as quiet as you can and think about Willow and Wise Old Tree. Imagine them together at the edge of the forest, by the shiny, shimmering lake.

Think about Willow, with her long branches full of curly green leaves. Now picture Wise Old Tree and his strong branches full of brown, green and yellow leaves. Picture his branches moving gently in the wind.

Staying quiet, look beyond Willow and Wise Old Tree.

Picture the large, shimmering lake in front of Willow. Imagine hearing the sounds of ducks moving and quacking on the lake and the sound of the water gently lapping against the bank.

Listen really hard.

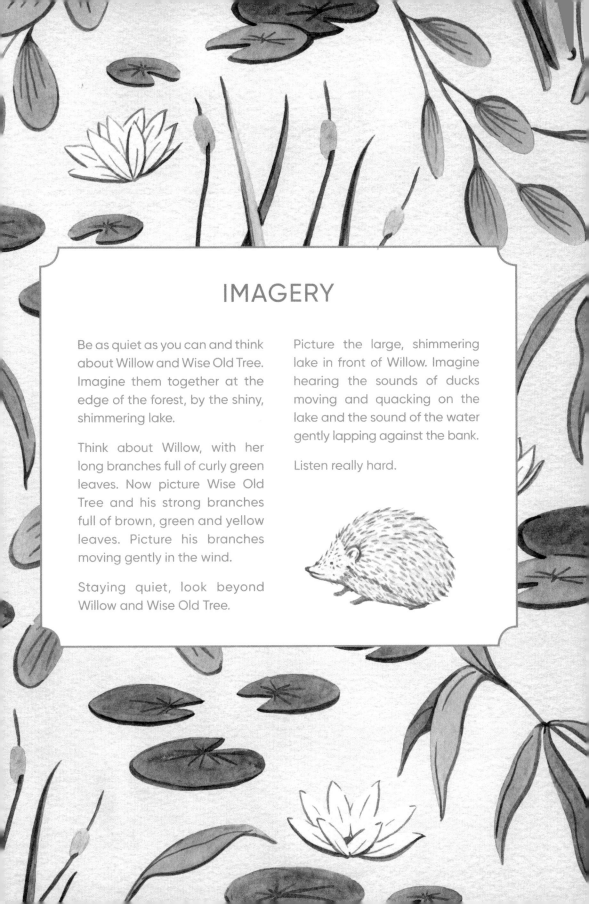

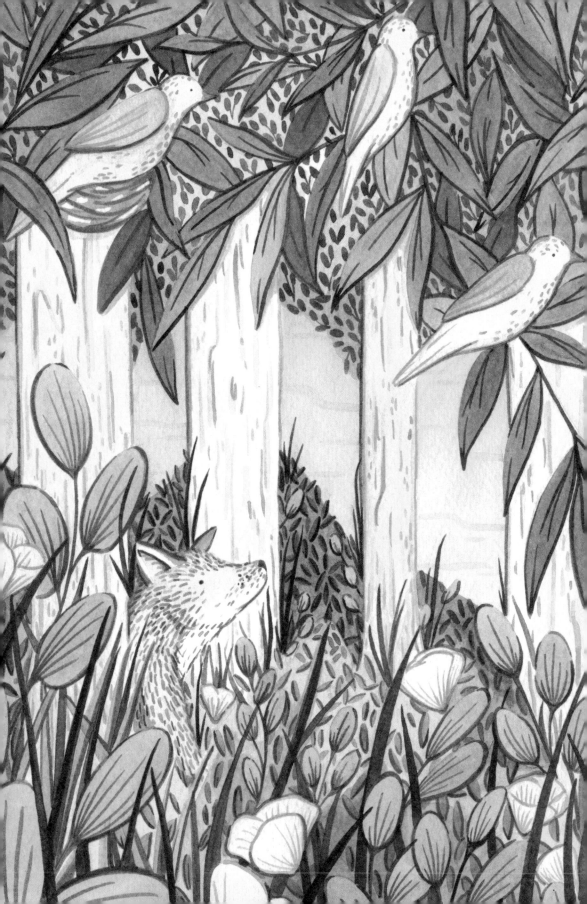

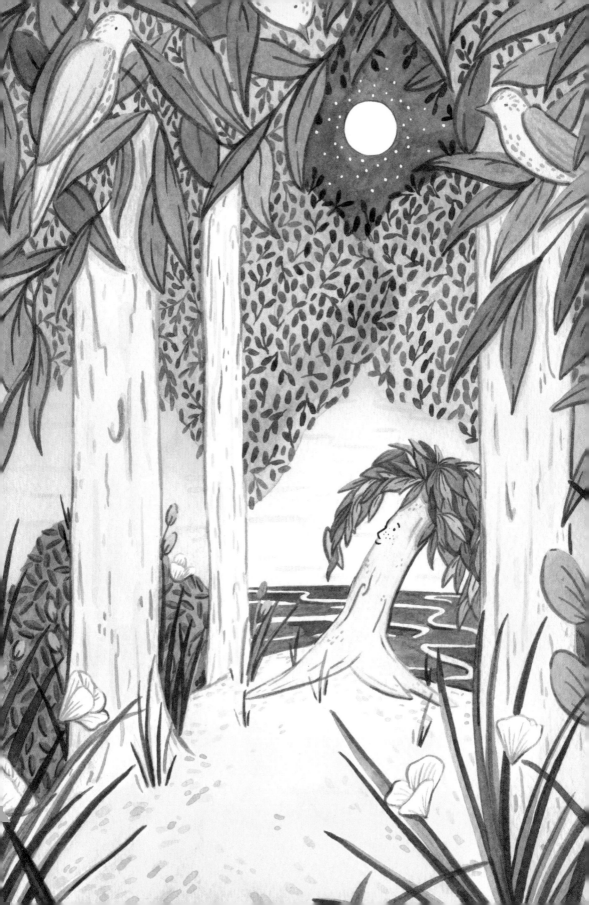

Willow thought Wise Old Tree was probably right, but she couldn't stop thinking about what happened at night-time. Every year, when Willow celebrated her birthday, she made a wish that she could stay up late and see what happened when she would normally be asleep.

Year after year, Willow made the same wish on her birthday. Then the day approached when she was no longer an infant, but was about to become a grown-up tree.

"What would you like for your birthday?" Wise Old Tree asked.

"I would really like to stay up past bedtime – just for a little bit – to see what happens in the forest at night-time," Willow replied thoughtfully.

"Very well," said Wise Old Tree. "When you are a grown-up, you must do what is right for you. But you know I won't be able to join you, as I always go to sleep at the same time each night. In fact, it's my bedtime now."

Wise Old Tree said goodnight and began to get ready for bed. He sleeps best when he rests on a bed of soft, warm soil.

Let's make the soil warm and soft for Wise Old Tree.

MUSCLE RELAXATION

Imagine you have some soil in your hands. Be quiet and lie very, very still. Be as calm and as quiet and as still as you can be.

First, let's squeeze your hands really hard, so that the soil gets soft and warm for Wise Old Tree. That's right, keep squeezing. The soil is becoming just right for Wise Old Tree's bed. Now relax your hands. Take a really big breath, in through your nose and out through your mouth.

Take a deep breath in … and a slow breath out… Relax for five, four, three, two, one. Feel how sleepy your hands are now.

Now it's time to squeeze the soil with your feet, so that the earth under your toes gets soft and warm too. Squeeze your feet. That's right, keep squeezing.

Now relax them.

Take a deep breath in … and a slow breath out… Relax for five, four, three, two, one. Feel how sleepy your feet are now.

Finally, let's squeeze the soil with your whole body. Keep squeezing the soil with every part of your body. That's right, keep squeezing. Now relax.

Take a deep breath in … and a slow breath out… Relax for five, four, three, two, one. Feel how relaxed your whole body is now.

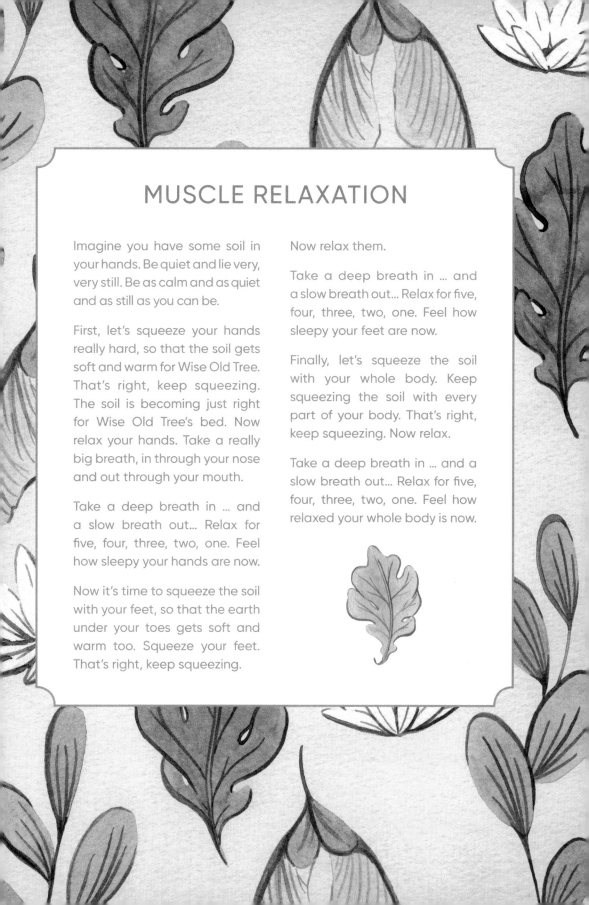

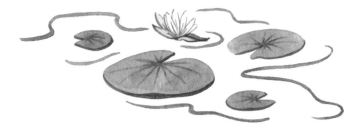

Well done. There is enough soft, warm soil to make a cosy bed that is perfect for Wise Old Tree to sleep on.

Although her birthday was only a few days later, the wait felt like forever. Finally, the big day arrived. Willow had a party and invited all the creatures of the forest. Deer and squirrels, ducks, swans, woodpeckers and all sorts of animals gathered by the edge of the lake to celebrate Willow's special day.

As the day grew late and the sun started to drop low behind the trees, the forest creatures began to rub their eyes and started gathering their families together, ready to return to their homes.

"Will anyone stay up with me, to see what happens in the forest at night-time?" Willow asked.

The forest animals smiled but shook their heads.

"Thanks, Willow, but we are all tired now," one of the deer told Willow. "I need my sleep to be ready for tomorrow. The fawn all get up as soon as the sun rises, and I need my energy to look after them!"

The other animals all told Willow why they too needed to get home to their warm, cosy beds.

"Never mind," Willow said. "I'll stay up on my own – just for a little while."

The forest creatures said their goodbyes and left to go home. Wise Old Tree wished Willow a very happy birthday and then he too went to bed. Willow felt the air grow cooler and the sky become darker. Before long, she couldn't see anything other than shadows and the only sound she could hear was the occasional swish of the leaves.

The owl, who is awake at night and asleep during the day, woke up and came out of a nearby tree. He was surprised to see Willow still awake.

"Aren't you tired?" the owl asked Willow. "It's very late."

Willow had to admit that she was getting just a little bit sleepy. Her branches were starting to droop, and her roots were getting tired.

"What happens in the forest at night?" Willow asked the owl. "That's what I really want to find out."

"Well," the owl told her, "it's hard for you to see, but there are other owls here and bats and other night-time creatures, all doing what they need to do while the day creatures sleep. Then, in the morning, we go to sleep and the day creatures get up."

Willow was really tired now. She looked at Wise Old Tree. He was fast asleep, getting his strength back for tomorrow.

"I think it's time for me to go to sleep, now, too," Willow told the owl, yawning. "I really am ... very ... sleepy."

Wise Old Tree was as wise as his name. There was a reason he went to bed at the same time each night. Now that Willow was a grown-up tree – well, she decided, she wouldn't stay up late after all. She would go to bed at the same time each night – at the very same time as Wise Old Tree.

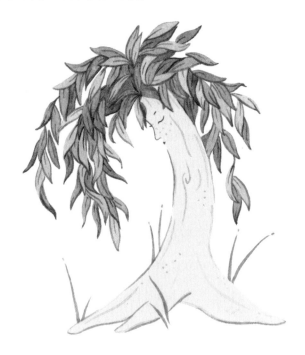

MINDFULNESS

Now it's time for *you* to close *your* eyes. For the next few minutes, you are going to relax and get all cosy and snug, just like Willow in her forest.

Try and get comfortable.

Choose a position that makes you feel relaxed. You could lie on your side or on your back. That's right, get really comfortable in your bed and relax.

Let your head rest on your pillow. Think really carefully about how your pillow feels under your head. Don't speak, but take a few moments to notice what is happening right here, right now. There is no right or wrong way to feel.

Staying quiet, think to yourself whether you feel hot or cold.

Let's think about your breathing now. You might feel air coming in through your nose when you breathe, or you may feel your tummy filling up like a balloon and then deflating.

Take a deep breath in.
Now slowly let it out.
Take a deep breath in.
Now let it out.

Take a deep breath in ...
and a slow breath out.
In ... and out...

Staying still, notice how your arms feel. They might feel tired or they might feel relaxed. There is no right or wrong way to feel.

Without moving, think carefully about how your legs feel. They might feel tired from running and moving all day, or they might feel rested.

Think about what is happening right here, right now. Feel the air coming into your tummy, and going out again.

Take a deep breath in ...
and a slow breath out.
In ... and out.

Let yourself sleep whenever you are ready.

Goodnight, Sleepy Tree.

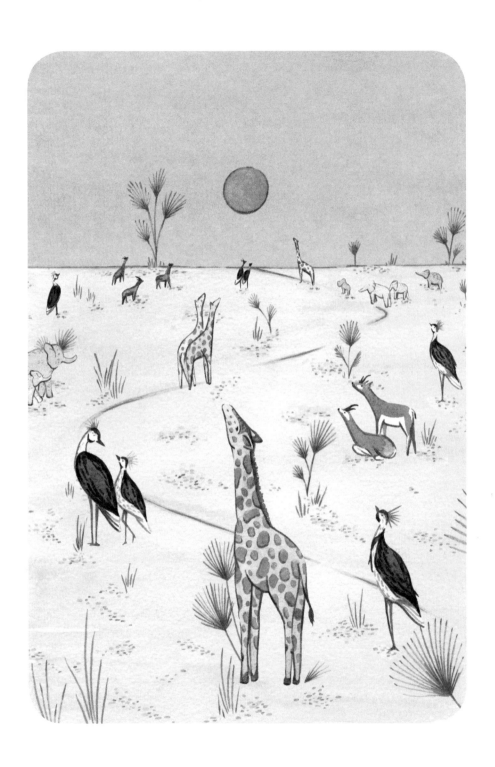

THE GIRAFFE WHO LIKED A BATH

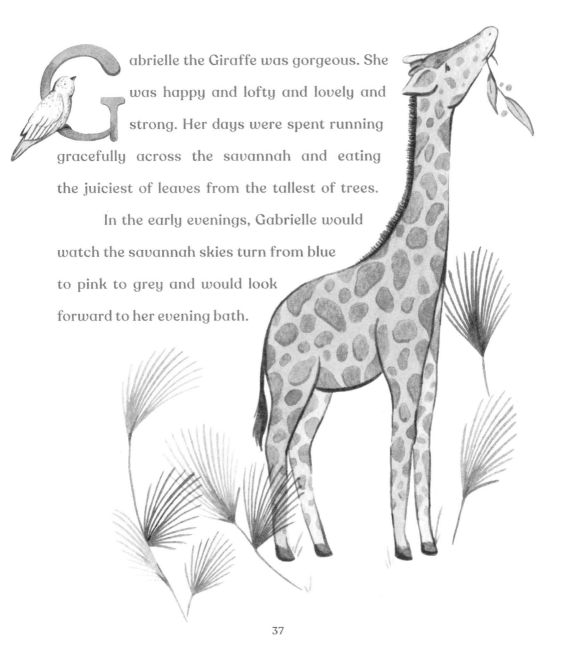

Gabrielle the Giraffe was gorgeous. She was happy and lofty and lovely and strong. Her days were spent running gracefully across the savannah and eating the juiciest of leaves from the tallest of trees.

In the early evenings, Gabrielle would watch the savannah skies turn from blue to pink to grey and would look forward to her evening bath.

When the sun was almost ready to disappear, Gabrielle would leave the other giraffes to join her friends, Ethel the Elephant and Hubert the Hippo. They would enjoy a long, relaxing soak in the water of the river. She was a giraffe who liked a bath.

Although Gabrielle loved her evening bath, she had one wish: she wished that her bath was deeper. She would watch Ethel and Hubert happily wallowing in the water, right up to their necks, but Gabrielle could only splash and paddle.

The other giraffes would laugh as she waded into the water, which barely reached her knees.

"A bath for a giraffe?" they asked every night, as they stood on the bank of the river licking themselves clean. "We've never heard of anything so strange!"

But Gabrielle just smiled and said the same thing each night:

"I'm a creature of habit and habit I like, I take a long bath to relax me at night."

Let's imagine Gabrielle in the river.

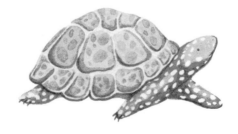

IMAGERY

Be as quiet as you can and think about Gabrielle in the river in the savannah. Try to picture her relaxing with her friends. Look beyond the river to see the other giraffes watching.

Think about the stars in the night sky. Imagine them shining brightly, and the dark sky behind them. Feel the slight chill in the air as day turns to night.

Now think about how quiet it is in the savannah at night-time.

Most of the animals are going to sleep now, and you can only hear the sound of the water flowing and the leaves moving softly in the breeze.

Listen really hard.

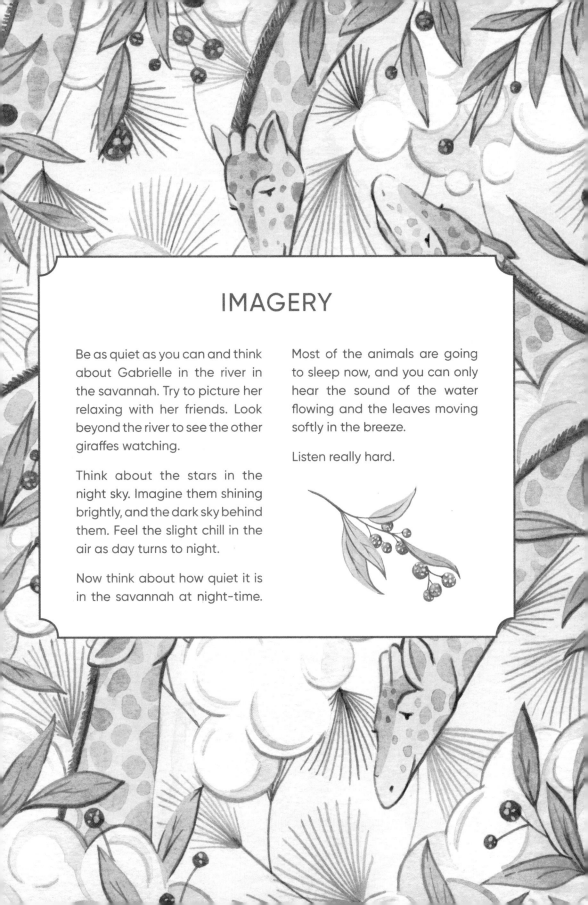

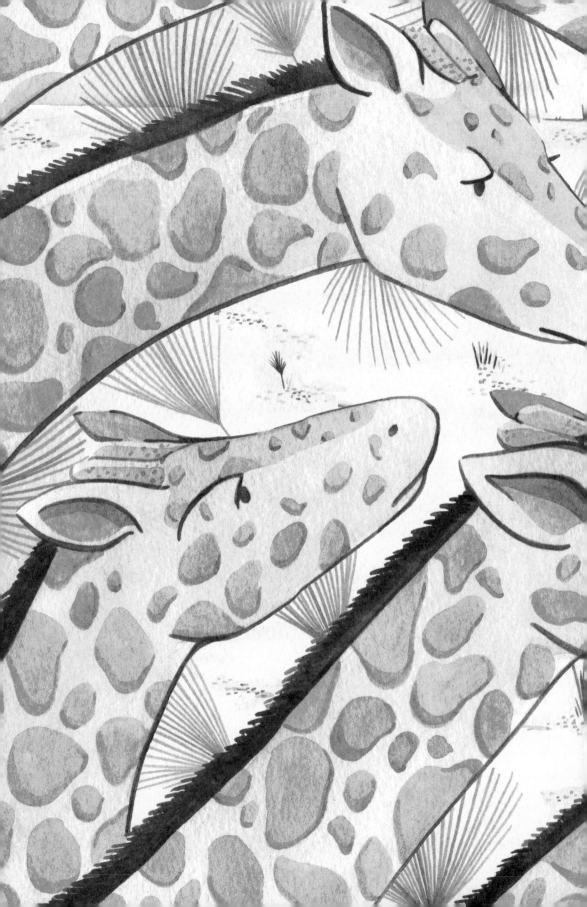

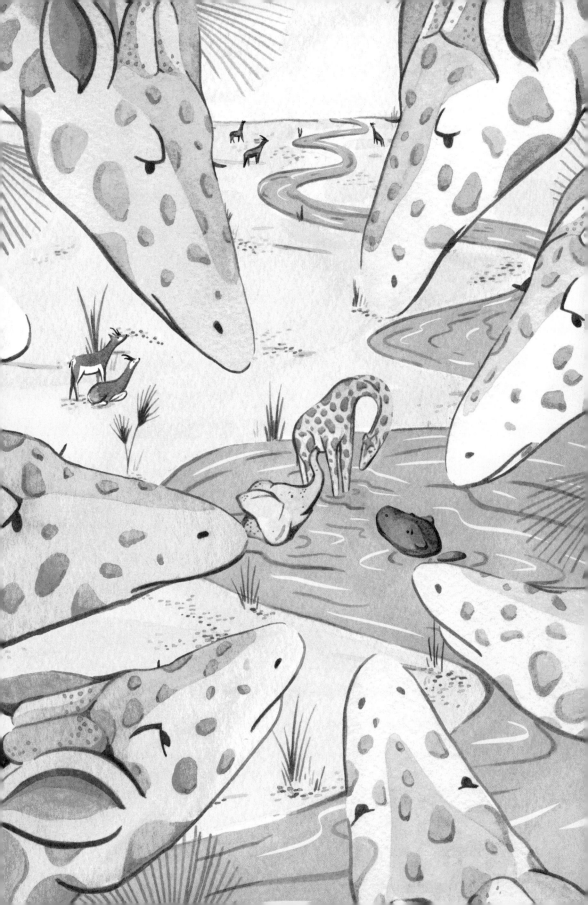

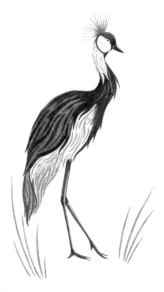

One day, Gabrielle had spent many hours craning her neck to reach the juiciest of leaves from the tallest of trees and thought again how lovely it would be to have a deep bath. She wanted the warm water to reach right up to the top of her neck – but it still only reached her knees.

"What's up?" Ethel asked when she saw Gabrielle's drooping eyelids and downturned mouth.

"I'm a creature of habit and habit I like,

*I would like a **deep** bath to relax me tonight."*

Ethel looked up at the sky. The clouds looked heavy. She had an idea.

Let's see if we can squeeze the clouds so that the rain falls down into the river and makes a deep bath for Gabrielle.

MUSCLE RELAXATION

Imagine that you can see the big, heavy clouds in the savannah. Be quiet and lie very still. Be as calm and as quiet and as still as you can be.

First, let's squeeze the clouds with both hands. Squeeze really tight so that the water comes out of them, like a sponge That's right, keep squeezing. It is starting to rain, and water is falling into the river. Now relax your hands.

Take a really big breath in through your nose and slowly out through your mouth. Take a deep breath in ... and a slow breath out... Relax for five, four, three, two, one. Feel how sleepy your hands are now.

Now it's time to squeeze the clouds with your feet, so that more rain will start to fall. Squeeze your feet. That's right, keep squeezing. Now relax them.

Take a deep breath in ... and a slow breath out... Relax for five, four, three, two, one. Feel how sleepy your feet are now.

Finally, let's squeeze the clouds with your whole body, so that the rain keeps falling and fills the river all the way up. Squeeze your body as tightly as you can, so that all the last raindrops are squeezed out of the clouds. The river is almost full. That's right, keep squeezing. Now relax.

Take a deep breath in ... and a slow breath out... Relax for five, four, three, two, one. Feel how relaxed your whole body is now.

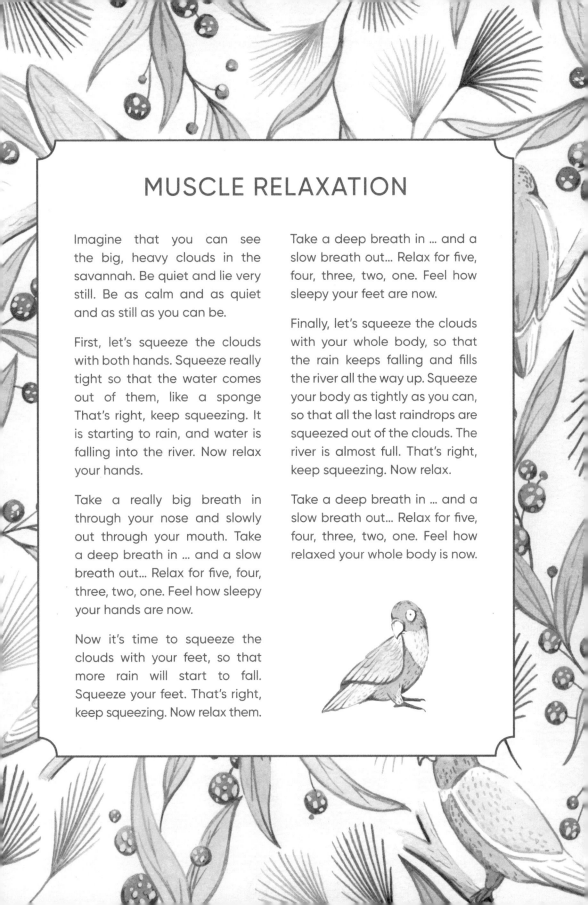

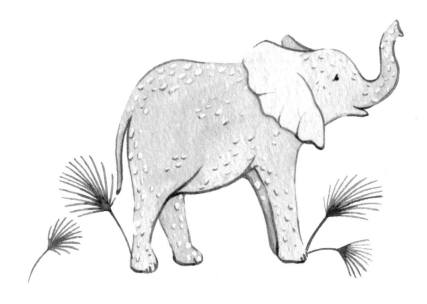

Well done. The river is full to the brim of fresh rainwater, ready for Gabrielle and her friends to have a relaxing, deep bath.

Gabrielle, Ethel and Hubert were very happy to have deep water for their baths. As she wallowed in the water, Gabrielle noticed that her long neck felt truly relaxed.

Before getting out of the river bath to join the other giraffes, Gabrielle told her friends how happy she was.

"I'm a creature of habit and habit I like,

*I enjoyed my **deep** bath that relaxed me tonight."*

Ethel and Hubert agreed. They were creatures of habit too, and they had loved their deep baths tonight.

Gabrielle, Ethel and Hubert looked up at the stars in the sky. It was time to go home to bed.

Gabrielle waded out of the water and settled down on a bed of grass with the other giraffes. She let her splendid neck rest. Her feet were weary from supporting her long, long legs, so she let them be still and peaceful. Her lashes pulled her eyelids shut.

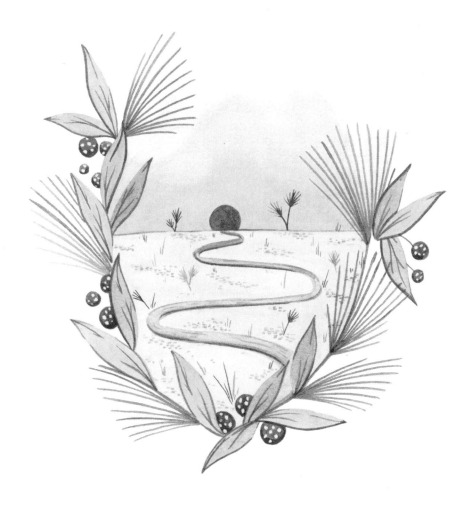

MINDFULNESS

Now it's time for *you* to close *your* eyes. For the next few minutes, you are going to relax and get all cosy and snug, just like Gabrielle in her grass.

Try and get comfortable.

Choose a position that makes you feel relaxed. You could lie on your side or on your back. That's right, get really comfortable in your bed and relax.

Let your head rest on your pillow. Think really carefully about how your pillow feels under your head. Don't speak, but take a few moments to notice what is happening right here, right now. There is no right or wrong way to feel.

Staying quiet, think to yourself whether you feel hot or cold.

Let's think about your breathing now. You might feel air coming in through your nose when you breathe, or you may feel your tummy filling up like a balloon and then deflating.

Take a deep breath in.
Now slowly let it out.
Take a deep breath in.
Now let it out.

Take a deep breath in ...
and a slow breath out.
In ... and out...

Staying still, notice how your arms feel. They might feel tired or they might feel relaxed. There is no right or wrong way to feel.

Without moving, think really carefully about how your legs feel. They might feel tired from running and moving all day, or they might feel rested.

Think about what is happening right here, right now. Feel the air coming into your tummy, and going out again.

Take a deep breath in ...
and a slow breath out.
In ... and out.

Let yourself sleep whenever you are ready.

Goodnight, Sleepy Giraffe.

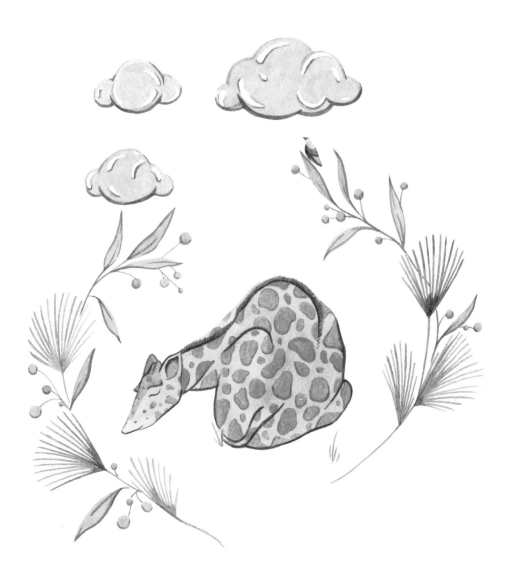

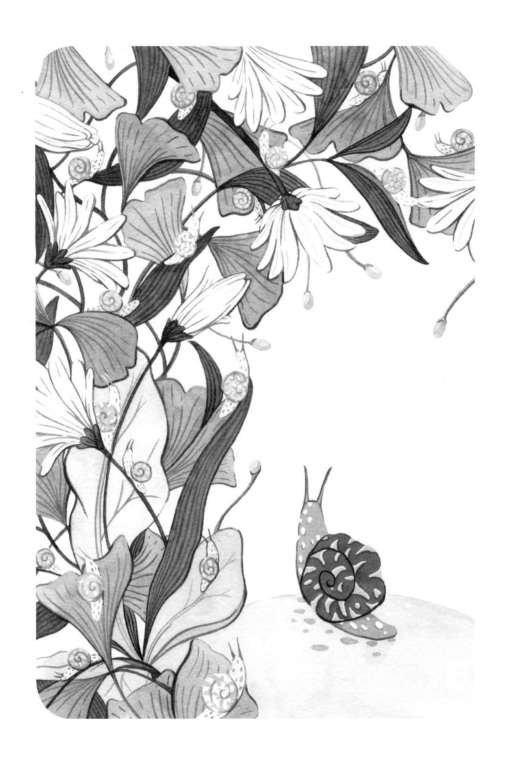

THE EVER-SO-TIRED SNAIL

Snails are slow and careful creatures. The snail we meet today has been slow and careful all his life. He has taken care of his children and he has taken care of his home, which is a snug shell that sits on his back.

Over the years, the colours on the snail's shell have faded and it is a strange shape now. It is no longer smooth, but it is lumpy and bumpy, bumpy and lumpy. But it is comfy, and it isn't too hot, it isn't too cold and it is lovely and dark at bedtime.

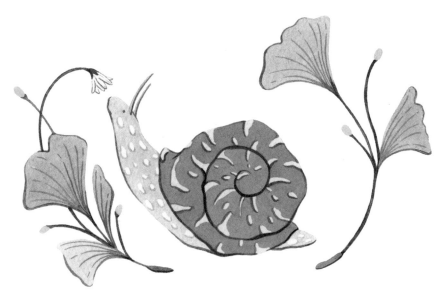

The snail is called Ernest. "I'm Ernest the snail, careful and kind," he used to tell his children, who have grown up now and have homes and children of their own.

Ernest is visiting his family today and he spends the day playing with his children and his children's children.

When the grandchildren curl up happily in their tiny shells for their after-lunch naps, Ernest's eldest son slides over to him.

"Dad," his son says, "I was thinking ... why don't I come over one day and give your shell a scrub? It has lost its colour now and it's a bit out of shape. It's looking a little bit..."

"...lovely," Ernest says, smiling. "The word you are looking for is 'lovely'. I have looked after my shell all my life. My shell is my home and my shell is my castle. My shell is so lovely for me."

At the end of the day, Ernest waves goodbye to his children and to his grandchildren, and starts making his way back to the leafy tree where he always sleeps at night.

Ernest is feeling weary now. He has been busy all day listening and chattering, chattering and listening and now he is looking forward to relaxing.

Let's imagine Ernest on his journey.

IMAGERY

Be as quiet as you can and think about Ernest the snail as he makes his way back to the tree where he spends his nights.

Think about the fading shell on his back. Be still and calm, and imagine the swirls and lines on the shell. Think about the dusty shades of brown and orange.

Now think about Ernest's smooth and shiny tentacles. They are drooping because Ernest is so weary.

Now imagine the feeling of the ground beneath Ernest. Some of it is smooth and some of it is lumpy and bumpy where there are stones.

Staying quiet, imagine the sky above Ernest. The sun is starting to set, so there are oranges and reds in the sky and a little bit of darkness. Picture the clouds in the sky and look at their shapes. See if you can picture the outline of the moon. Listen to the sound of the trees.

Listen really hard.

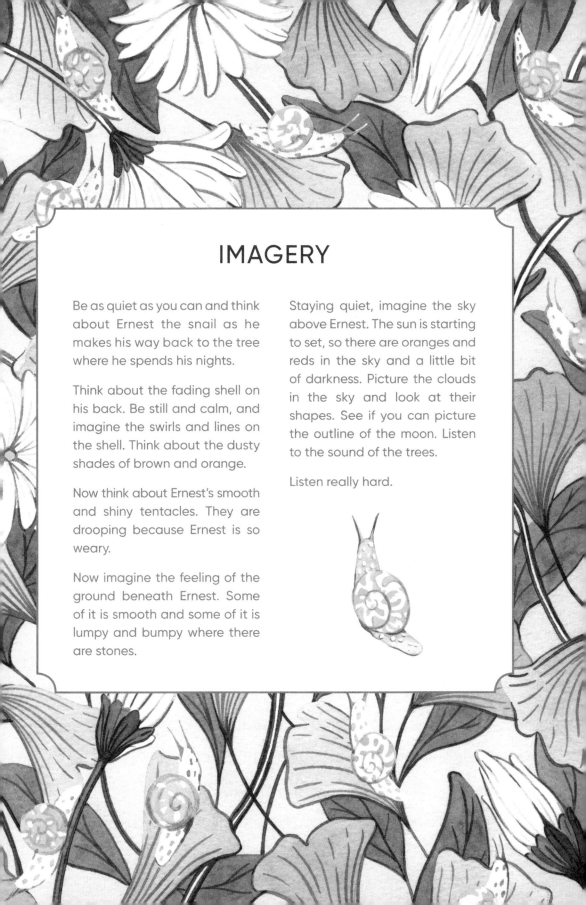

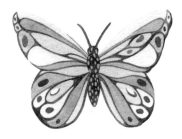

Ernest is always slow and careful, but he is starting to move even more slowly and carefully than usual. It takes a lot of effort to keep moving forwards, and his shell feels heavy on his back. He stops and rests for a minute.

Ernest feels a raindrop tap on his shell, then another and then another. Before long, the raindrops are coming quickly and it's hard to see the path ahead. Ernest lowers his tentacles and hopes the rain will pass.

An earwig, asleep in a fallen branch, wakes to the sound of the rain. He pokes his head out and sees Ernest.

"Are you OK?" the earwig asks, yawning, and looking at Ernest. "You must be getting wet. Your shell looks a bit..."

"Lovely," Ernest says, although it's hard to hear him with the noise of the raindrops splashing against the ground. "The word you are looking for is 'lovely'. I have looked after my shell all my life. My shell is my home and my shell is my castle. My shell is so lovely for me."

The rain keeps falling harder and faster, faster and harder, so the earwig shrugs and sighs and scurries back into the shelter of his fallen branch.

Ernest moves slowly through the rain, making his way to the side of the path. There are some shrubs there that keep him a little bit dryer and stop the rain from beating down on his face while he rests. He feels something, or someone, watching him and looks up.

A spider, with long, thin legs and a wide, lazy smile, is lounging on a leaf.

"Hi," says the spider.

"Hello," says Ernest.

"Do you want to climb up here and sit with me?" the spider asks, stretching and yawning, yawning and stretching. "It's dry and we can chat for a while."

"No, thank you," Ernest says. "I'm very tired and would fall asleep straight away."

"Well, that's OK," says the spider. "Why don't you come and sleep here anyway? It's dry up here. Your shell looks kind of..."

"Lovely," Ernest says. "The word you are looking for is 'lovely'. I have looked after my shell all my life. My shell is my home and my shell is my castle. My shell is so lovely for me."

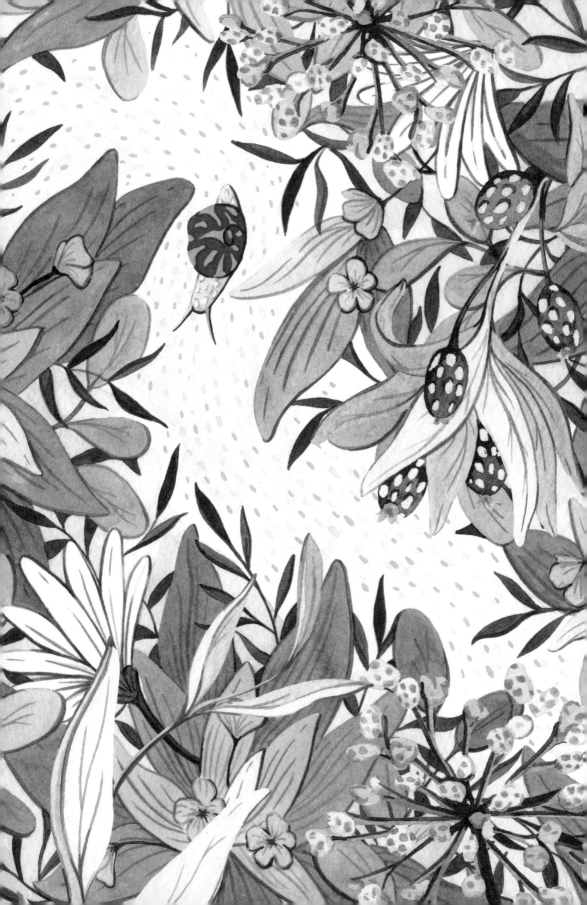

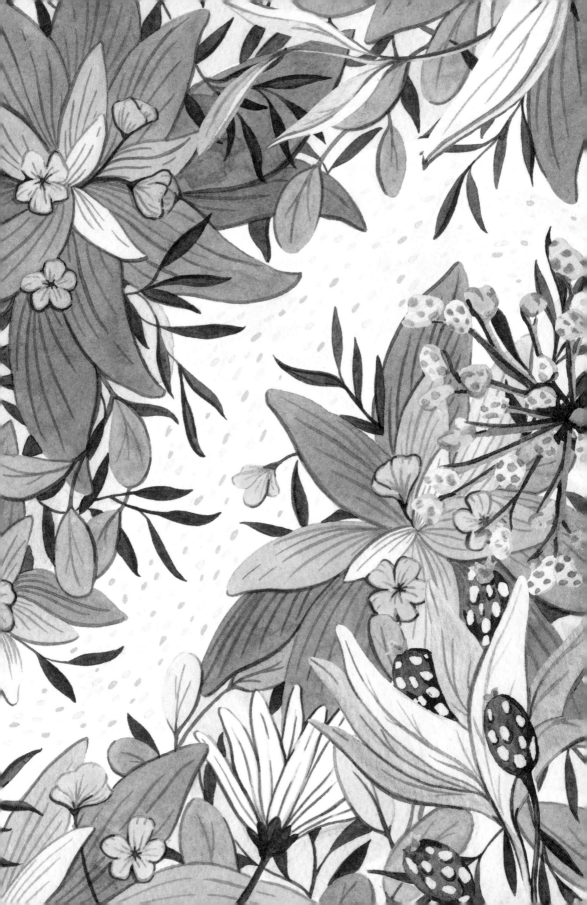

"OK," the spider shrugs. "I'm here if you change your mind."

Ernest is still tired after his rest, but he keeps thinking about his leafy tree. He decides to set off again and keep moving until he reaches it, however long it takes. He moves very slowly now. Ernest is ever so tired ... so weary ... and so ready to sleep.

Ernest keeps moving forwards, and as he does, the rain eases a little until it is just a gentle patter. The sky grows darker and darker and the moon comes out. Finally, shining in the light of the moon, Ernest sees his leafy tree.

Ernest is very happy to be back at the leafy tree as it's nearly bedtime. He reads a story about the adventures of three friends – a tortoise, a sloth and a slug.

Let's help Ernest get ready for bed.

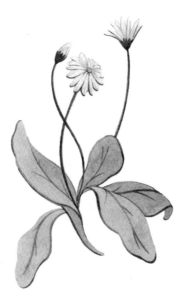

MUSCLE RELAXATION

Imagine that you are Ernest, feeling tired and getting ready to squeeze your whole body into your shell, which is your home and your castle. Be quiet and lie very, very still. Be as calm and as quiet and as still as you can be.

First, get your hands ready to squeeze into your shell. Squeeze them into a tiny ball. That's right, keep squeezing. Now relax your hands.

Take a really big breath, in through your nose and slowly out through your mouth. Take a deep breath in ... and a slow breath out... Relax for five, four, three, two, one. Feel how sleepy your hands are now.

Now it's time to squeeze your feet, so that they can fit right into the lumps and bumps of your shell. Squeeze your feet.

That's right, keep squeezing. Now relax them.

Take a deep breath in ... and a slow breath out... Relax for five, four, three, two, one. Feel how sleepy your feet are now.

Finally, let's squeeze your whole body into the shell. Tense all your muscles as hard as you can. That's right, keep squeezing. Now relax.

Take a deep breath in ... and a slow breath out... Relax for five, four, three, two, one. Feel how relaxed your whole body is now.

Well done. Ernest fits into his shell beautifully.

Ernest is safe and snug. It is quiet in his shell. It is dark. It is not too hot and it is not too cold. He starts to fall asleep, relaxed in his shell-bed. As he falls asleep, he thinks about how lucky he is to have such a cosy, comfy place to sleep.

"People might think my shell is old and shabby," Ernest whispers to himself sleepily, "but it is so perfect for me. I have looked after it all my life. My shell is my home, and my shell is my castle. My shell is so lovely for me."

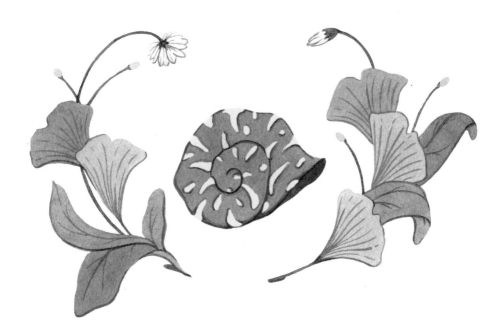

MINDFULNESS

Now it's time for *you* to close *your* eyes. For the next few minutes, you are going to relax and get all cosy and snug, just like Ernest the snail.

Try and get comfortable.

Choose a position that makes you feel relaxed. You could lie on your side or on your back. That's right, get really comfortable in your bed and relax.

Let your head rest on your pillow. Think really carefully about how your pillow feels under your head. Don't speak, but take a few moments to notice what is happening right here, right now. There is no right or wrong way to feel.

Staying quiet, think to yourself whether you feel hot or cold.

Let's think about your breathing now. You might feel air coming in through your nose when you breathe, or you may feel your tummy filling up like a balloon and then deflating.

Take a deep breath in.
Now slowly let it out.
Take a deep breath in.
Now let it out.

Take a deep breath in...
and a slow breath out.
In ... and out...

Staying still, notice how your arms feel. They might feel tired or they might feel relaxed. There is no right or wrong way to feel.

Without moving, think really carefully about how your legs feel. They might feel tired from running and moving all day, or they might feel rested.

Think about what is happening right here, right now. Feel the air coming into your tummy, and going out again.

Take a deep breath in...
and a slow breath out.
In ... and out.

Let yourself sleep whenever you are ready.

Goodnight, Sleepy Snail.

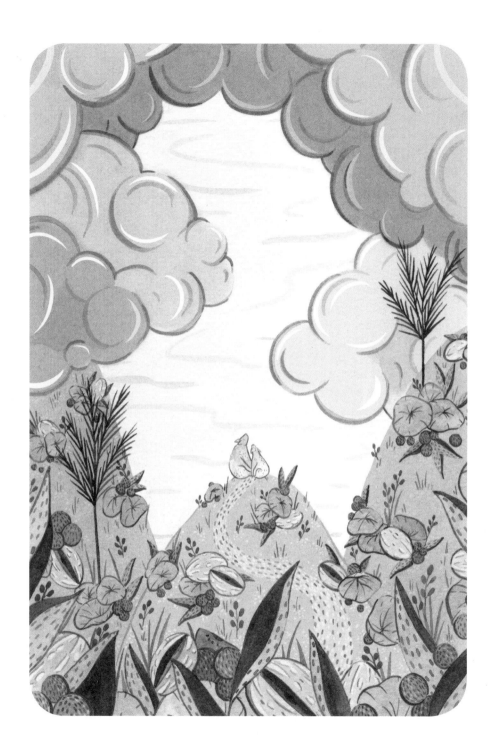

THE PIG WHO NEEDED TO SLEEP

Paul was a splendid pot-bellied pig. He was not much bigger than a cat, and he was bristly and handsome too. He had the littlest legs and a tummy that sagged so low that it almost scraped the ground. He lived with his Great Pig Ma in the mountains.

Let's think about Paul the pig.

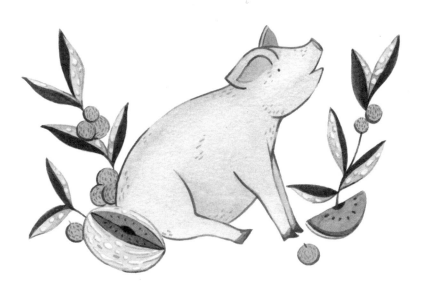

IMAGERY

Be as quiet as you can and think about Paul on his mountain. Imagine the clouds touching the mountain tops and casting long shadows.

Think about Paul sitting with his Great Pig Ma. Think about his rough skin covered with some bristly hair. Imagine gently stroking his little head.

Now think about the mountain. Picture a gravel path winding up the mountain and imagine a patch of grass in shades of green and brown. Think about the green trees and plants all around. Think about breathing in the lovely fresh air.

Staying quiet, look up at the blue sky above. There are fluffy clouds scattered throughout. Listen to the sound of the breeze.

Listen really hard.

Paul was a happy little pig – but never happier than when he was cooking. Ever since he was a young piglet, Paul had loved cooking and eating. Great Pig Ma was a talented chef, and he spent as much time as he could learning from her and helping in the kitchen.

Each year, Great Pig Ma hosted a Great Feast for all the animals of the mountain. She would select one of her young to cook food for the feast. So far, every one of his brothers and sisters had been asked, but Paul had not. He always dreamed of being asked to cook at the Great Feast himself, but the day never seemed to arrive.

Then one day, just before the feast, Great Pig Ma turned to him with a smile.

"Now it is your go, to cook a feast solo," she said.

Paul leapt for joy.

"Oh, thank you!" he said with a smile so wide that you could hardly see his kind little eyes.

Paul sprang into action and spent the day foraging and collecting seeds. He chopped, mashed and beat, sieved, mixed and baked.

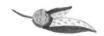

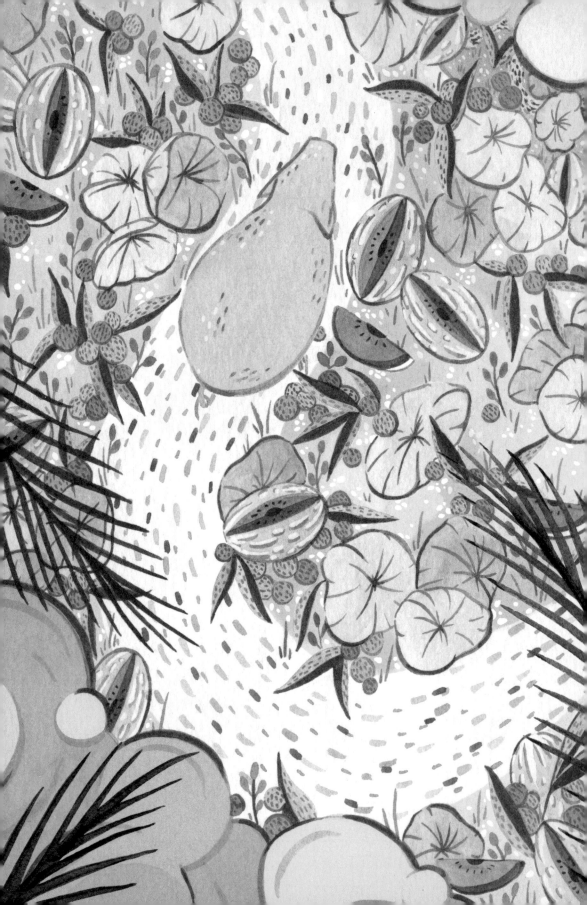

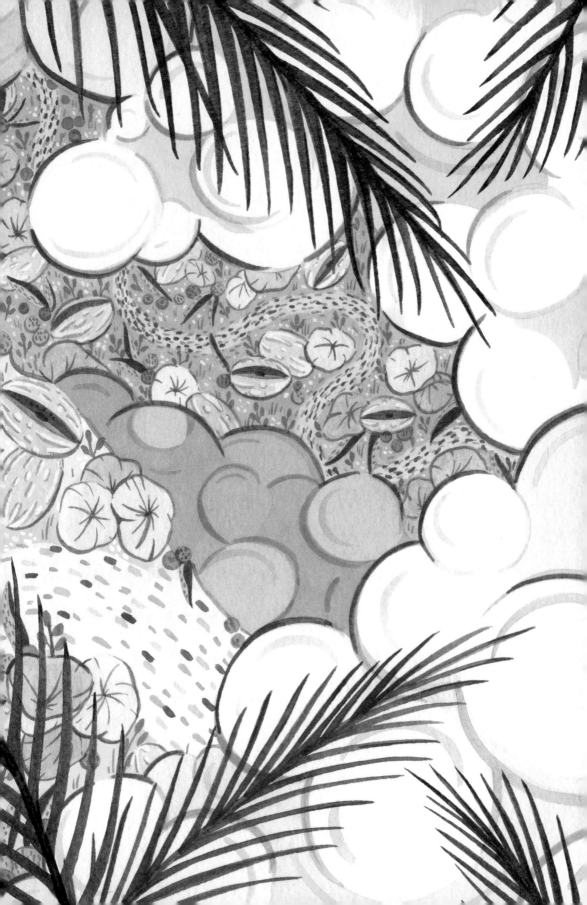

Finally, he produced a feast so incredible that every animal on the mountain would talk about it for years to come. Yet there was still one item left to make. He had not yet finished making his seed bread, which was to be his tastiest dish.

"Have you finished your seed bread? asked Great Pig Ma.

"Not yet!" said Paul. "Today my dough is low. It just won't seem to grow."

Great Pig Ma went over to look at the seed bread. The dough did look a bit flat.

"You must knead the dough so it can rise," said Great Pig Ma.

Let's help Paul to knead his dough.

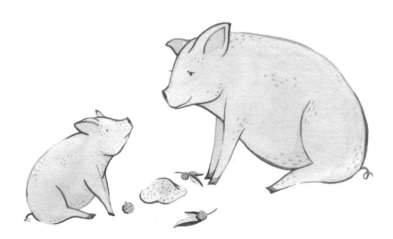

MUSCLE RELAXATION

Imagine you have some warm, soft dough in your hands. Be quiet and lie very, very still as you get ready to knead the dough. Be as calm as you can.

First, squeeze your hands as tightly as you can, squeezing all the dough between your fingers. That's right, keep squeezing. The dough is becoming very soft. Now relax your hands.

Take a really big breath in through your nose and slowly out through your mouth. Take a deep breath in ... and a slow breath out... Relax for five, four, three, two, one. Feel how sleepy your hands are now.

Now, it's time to squeeze the dough with your toes. Squeeze them really hard, so that the dough will rise. Squeeze your feet. That's right, keep squeezing. Now relax them.

Take a deep breath in ... and a slow breath out... Relax for five, four, three, two, one. Feel how sleepy your feet are now.

Finally, let's squeeze the dough by tensing all your muscles as hard as you can. That means making all your muscles as strong as you can. Squeeze them really hard! Make your body feel really strong. That's right, keep squeezing. Now relax.

Take a deep breath in ... and a slow breath out... Relax for five, four, three, two, one. Feel how relaxed your whole body is now.

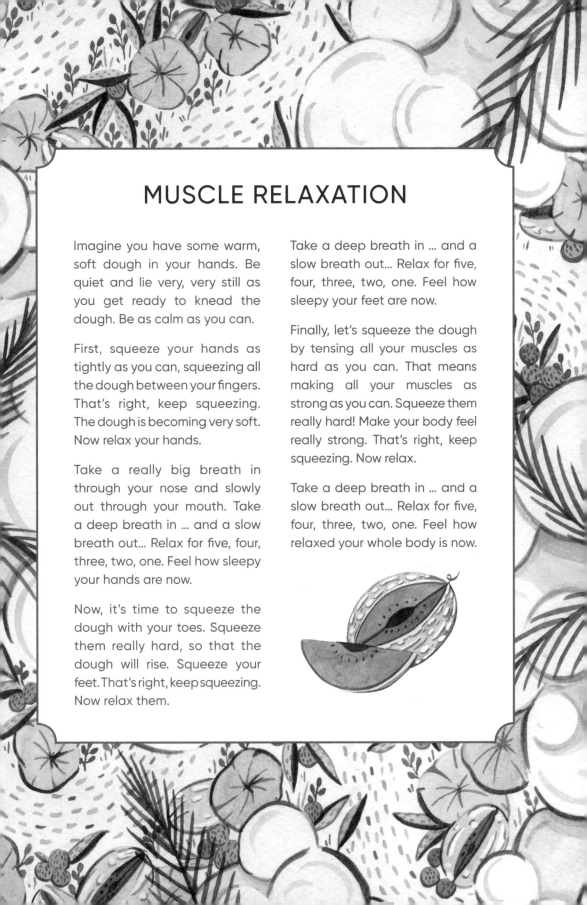

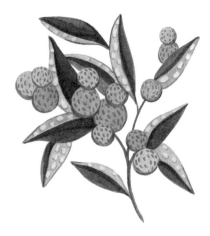

Well done. The dough has been kneaded and it is ready to rise.

The dough looked wonderful. Once the bread was cooked, Paul and Great Pig Ma called for the other animals to come and eat and everyone enjoyed the tasty and colourful delights. Great Pig Ma and the other animals cheered for Paul, who they called the Greatest Chef in the Land.

Once the last animal had finished the final mouthful and left, Paul lay down on his side for a rest.

"Are you OK?" asked Great Pig Ma with a proud smile.

"I'm fine; I just feel slow. My tummy seems full and low."

Great Pig Ma thought for a while.

"Well, you have been tasting and testing all the roots, berries and seeds that you needed for the Great Feast," she said. "When night-time arrives, sleep will give your tummy time to rest and help you to turn your food into energy."

Paul thought this was marvellous. He liked the idea of food turning into energy.

Paul gave a big yawn.

"Are you tired?" asked Great Pig Ma.

"I am quite tired. My head and brain feel slow; my thoughts don't seem to flow," said Paul.

Great Pig Ma thought for a while.

"Well, you have been thinking about your recipes all day," she said. "It's no wonder your brain is tired."

Great Pig Ma looked up at the sky and saw the sun disappear behind a mountain top.

"It's almost night-time," she said, "you can go to bed soon to rest your weary head. Sleep can help you learn and remember things. When you wake up in the morning you might have good ideas for new and exciting treats for all your friends."

Paul stopped and thought about this for a while. He did like the idea of sleeping and resting his head, which felt very tired now.

"What's more," said Great Pig Ma, "sleep can help you grow, just like the marvellous seed bread you made earlier. You can grow tall and strong. So many things become better when you sleep."

Paul stopped and thought about this for a while. It was true that he wished he was a little taller and that his legs were stronger, so they did not feel so tired from trotting around all day.

Paul decided it was a very good idea to go to sleep, but as it was not quite bedtime, he decided to spend the last part of his day remembering the wonderful Great Feast that he had shared with his friends and thinking about how happy he was. Then, he got cosy in his bed and closed his eyes.

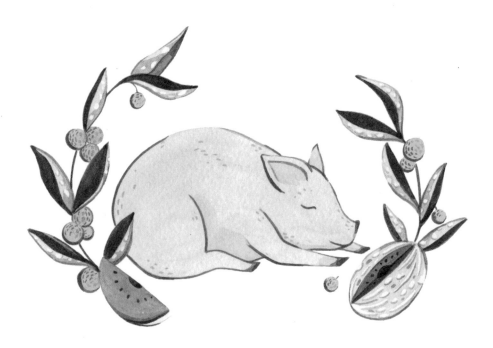

MINDFULNESS

Now it's time for *you* to close *your* eyes. For the next few minutes, you are going to relax and get all cosy and snug, just like Paul in his bed.

Try and get comfortable.

Choose a position that makes you feel relaxed. You could lie on your side or on your back. That's right, get really comfortable in your bed and relax.

Let your head rest on your pillow. Think really carefully about how your pillow feels under your head. Don't speak, but take a few moments to notice what is happening right here, right now. There is no right or wrong way to feel.

Staying quiet, think to yourself whether you feel hot or cold.

Let's think about your breathing now. You might feel air coming in through your nose when you breathe, or you may feel your tummy filling up like a balloon and then deflating.

Take a deep breath in.
Now slowly let it out.
Take a deep breath in.
Now let it out.

Take a deep breath in ...
and a slow breath out.
In ... and out...

Staying still, notice how your arms feel. They might feel tired or they might feel relaxed. There is no right or wrong way to feel.

Without moving, think really carefully about how your legs feel. They might feel tired from running and moving all day, or they might feel rested.

Think about what is happening right here, right now. Feel the air coming into your tummy, and going out again.

Take a deep breath in ...
and a slow breath out.
In ... and out.

Let yourself sleep whenever you are ready.

Goodnight, Sleepy Piggy.

TIPS FOR A RELAXING BEDTIME AND BETTER SLEEP

You may have received multiple tips to help make bedtime a more positive experience or to improve sleep for you and your child. Some tips that have a scientific basis or have been supported by literature are outlined here. Of course, every family is unique and you will have to decide whether or not a tip is helpful for you.

1. Think about your diet

Lots of food is lauded as soporific – from warm milk to tart cherries. There is some logic to some of these suggestions, as certain foods naturally contain substances that give our bodies a cue that it is time to fall asleep, such as melatonin (the 'darkness hormone'). It is currently unclear whether eating these foods can have a noteworthy impact on our sleep. Instead, the focus of our diet should be on what to avoid. Caffeine is a key example and can affect our sleep for prolonged periods after it is consumed. While it is unlikely that children will be drinking coffee, remember that caffeine is contained in multiple other foods such as cola and chocolate too – so these should also be avoided.

2. Be cool

Our core body temperature naturally drops before bedtime and a comfortably cool environment is conducive for good sleep. This may seem at odds with a desire for a warm bath before bed, but it is not. When we have a pleasantly warm bath, the blood vessels in our skin dilate which means that blood moves to the surface of our skin. When we leave the bath, the cool air lowers our blood temperature and we lose heat.

3. Dim the lights

When it gets dark, our bodies release the 'darkness hormone' melatonin. This gives our bodies a cue that it is time to go to sleep. Bright light can disrupt this process, so can potentially hamper a natural descent into sleep. Therefore, when you start to think about putting your child to bed, reduce light as much as you can by using blinds and curtains, dimming the light and avoiding electronic devices that emit light.

4. Remember the basic rules of shaping behaviour

A basic rule of shaping behaviour is to reinforce that which we like. We need to make sure that we do not accidentally reinforce behaviours which we do not appreciate. For example, if you would prefer your child to stay in bed at night – perhaps use a sticker chart to reward each night they do so. If your child gets up during the night without a good reason, don't reward this behaviour by allowing them play or have fun with those who are still awake.

5. Be clock-like

Our physiological processes are controlled by 'clocks' within our bodies. For example, our body temperature, melatonin secretion and alertness levels naturally change throughout the day and night. This means that at certain times of day we are more prepared for sleep than at others. If we keep our bedtime and wake time consistent, we help our body know when sleep is coming and to prepare accordingly.

6. Get an early night...

Certain guidelines suggest that most children aged between 3 and 5 years should get between 10 and 13 hours of sleep per 24 hours, whereas those aged between 6 and 13 should get between 9 and 11 hours. Many children do not get enough sleep, which can cause problems during the day. A good way to ensure that your child gets the sleep required is to get an early night. Wake time is often fixed (we need to get up for work or school) and perhaps unsurprisingly, research has found that children who go to bed earlier get more sleep.

7. ...But not too early!

We should only go to bed when we are tired. If that does not happen, we may lie in bed unable to sleep. This can escalate into a sleep problem if we then start to associate being in bed with feeling awake and stressed. It can be confusing for parents to decide when their children are tired, as in contrast to most adults, children can sometimes behave in an excitable way when they are exhausted. You might want to try a given bedtime for a week or so in order to get the feel for whether that is just right for them, or whether they might need to go to bed earlier or later. Don't forget that sleep requirements change as children grow older, too.

8. No electronics

A large proportion of children have electronics in their bedroom. These can include a whole range of devices from tablets to mobile phones. Such devices often emit 'blue light' which is particularly disruptive to our bodies' ability to secrete the hormone melatonin – which means that our body may miss out on a cue to fall asleep. A 'night setting' on these devices can often be activated, but even in these alternative modes, electronic devices can be exciting (they might emit noise for example) and can lead to arousal before bedtime. Ideally, turn off such devices many hours before bedtime and keep them out of the bedroom.

9. Don't let sleep be bad or sad

For adults, going to bed is often a treat. It would be wonderful if children felt the same – so we should try to avoid sleep becoming something bad or sad. For example, it's not a good idea to tell your child that 'they must go to bed' if they do something wrong, or 'they can stay up late' as a reward for good behaviour. This reinforces the idea that being asleep is a punishment and being awake is a treat. Try to avoid conflating sleep and death, too. Avoid telling your child that someone who has died is 'at rest' or 'sleeping' as this can make sleep a frightening experience.

10. Enjoy the tranquillity of the bedroom

Research suggests that people report better sleep in fresh sheets and that air quality is important for good quality sleep. Avoid stress at night too! Although bedtime can be stressful, tension around this time can influence levels of the stress hormone cortisol and does not aid good sleep, so do all that you can to avoid it. Make your expectations about your child's behaviour and sleep clear well before bedtime and by showing consistency in your approach over time. However much you are challenged by your child, try to stay calm – making sure you do not raise your voice.

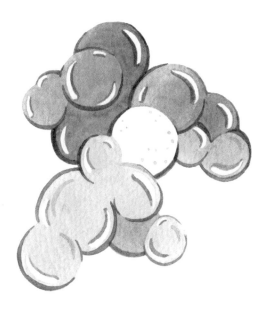

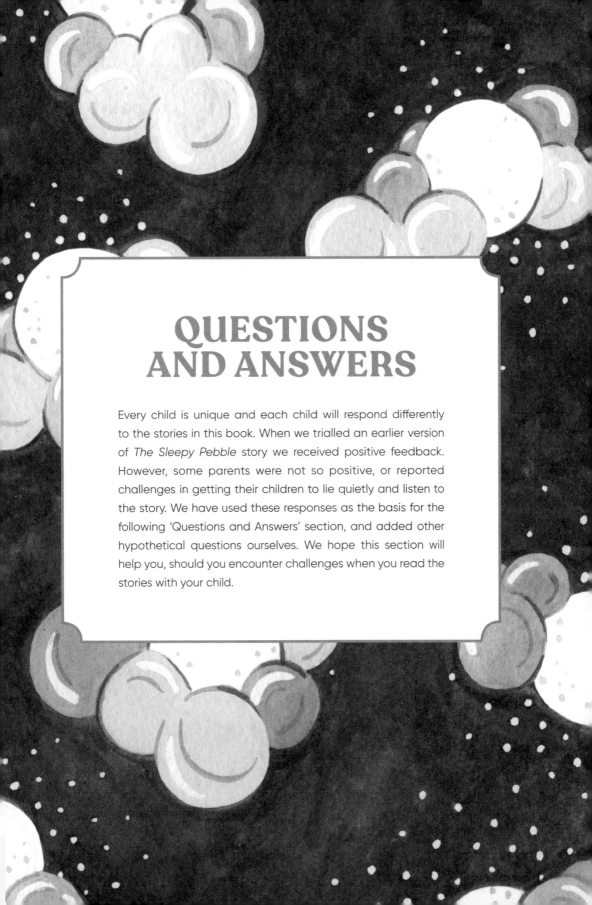

QUESTIONS
AND ANSWERS

Every child is unique and each child will respond differently to the stories in this book. When we trialled an earlier version of *The Sleepy Pebble* story we received positive feedback. However, some parents were not so positive, or reported challenges in getting their children to lie quietly and listen to the story. We have used these responses as the basis for the following 'Questions and Answers' section, and added other hypothetical questions ourselves. We hope this section will help you, should you encounter challenges when you read the stories with your child.

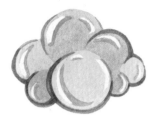

How old does my child need to be to use this book?

In our pilot study, a story from this book was read to children between 3 and 11 years of age. This book was reported to have a positive effect on sleep for children of varying ages, but not for all children. Certain components of these stories will likely have a different impact on children of different ages. For example, a 5-year-old will not be able to take part in imagery tasks in the same way as an 11-year-old, but may benefit from mindfulness (a technique which has been used with preschoolers). Feel free to alter or omit sections which you do not consider to be age-appropriate for your child.

My child has sleep problems. Can I use this book instead of seeking expert advice?

This book is not intended to replace medical advice. If your child is experiencing problems with their sleep, we would recommend starting by talking to your healthcare provider.

My child does not want to lie down or be still. What should I do?

Do all you can to create a calm environment at bedtime (see pages 73-77 for guidance about how to achieve this). However, on the first few occasions that your child is listening to the book, they may prefer to look at the pictures and ask questions about the story. Subsequently, you could explain that this is a book that will help them relax and encourage quietness and stillness while they are listening to it. It is important to avoid conflict before bed, so if your child doesn't want to lie down and would prefer to listen to the book sitting up, that is fine. You might want to agree that your child is still for the relaxation sections. If on a certain night your child is particularly fidgety and you do not feel they are responsive to the story, choose a book that they do want to read. You might want to try again another night.

I have more than one child and the children become excitable when they are in a room together. How can I manage this situation?

If it is possible to stagger bedtime so that each child hears the story on their own, this could help prevent children from making each other excitable. However, if this is not possible (e.g. you have a child who cannot be left unattended), try to keep the bedtime routine as calm as possible, by following the advice on pages 73-77 of this book. Explain that they should try to ignore what other children might be doing during the story, too.

My child is not fully engaged in the stories or sleep techniques. Should I continue to read the story to them?

Explain to your child that this is a story to help them relax, so it might not seem as exciting as other stories they read. More exciting stories can come earlier in the day or evening. If your child does not enjoy one particular story in the book, they might enjoy a different story instead. However, if the story or any of the sleep techniques embedded in them makes them unsettled, stop reading.

My child is not going to sleep any quicker than they were before we started reading the story. Should I continue to read the book to them at bedtime?

If your child is enjoying the book you can keep reading the stories at bedtime even if you find that it doesn't help them relax. It may be that it takes a few nights for a child to become used to a particular story and for the techniques to be effective. Children's sleep can change from night to night, but if you feel that this book is unhelpful, discontinue use.

Do I have to use the different techniques exactly as they are listed in this book?

We developed and refined the techniques in this book based on our target ages and the feedback we received from families and experts in the field. However, you may prefer to adapt them to suit the specific child you are reading to. Some parents may want to explain unfamiliar words to their child or substitute them for other words if they think that would be beneficial. Older children might appreciate more details when imaging scenes (e.g. during *The Sleepy Pebble* you could ask them to taste the salt on their lips). Younger children might prefer less imagery. We have tried to keep the muscle relaxation sections short, but you could certainly add in relaxation of more parts of the body for older children (tensing and relaxing the face or shoulders for example) or remove some steps if it feels long. Some parents may want to embed the techniques flagged here into their own stories.

My child wants to know more about the story and why they are being asked to use these sleep techniques. What should I say?

It's great if your child is interested in the science behind the sleep techniques. Depending on the age and understanding of your child, you could spend some time with them in the daytime, or before you start reading the story, talking about the techniques and the importance of allowing your body and mind to relax before bedtime. When you start reading the story though, and especially after you have read the story to them a few times, try to encourage them to be quiet and still and to listen to the story.

My child looks at the pictures in the book instead of relaxing. How can I encourage them to close their eyes?

Your child may initially want to see all of the illustrations in the book. Once they have been read the stories a few times, you might want to encourage them to close their eyes as the story progresses. The book has been illustrated with the aim of keeping children calm, instead of exciting them.

My child finds the stories too long. What can I do?

Using this book is not intended to prolong bedtime. Instead, you may want to reduce other aspects of your bedtime routine (e.g. replace another bedtime story with this book). Some stories are longer than others, with *The Pig Who Needed to Sleep* being the shortest and *The Ever-So-Tired Snail* being the longest. It is fine to reduce sections if you feel they are too long for your child.

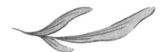

Acknowledgements

First, we'd like to thank Sam Arthur for being so enthusiastic about this project from the start, for pairing the authors and illustrator and for his invaluable help throughout. Thanks too to Joanna McInerney for her excellent editing and to everyone else at Nobrow. We are particularly grateful to the many experts (sleep scientists and clinicians, clinical psychologists, medical doctors, mindfulness experts and others) for providing inspiration or for their invaluable insight and feedback on this project. These include, but are not limited to, Drs Candice Alfano, Daniel Buysse, Catherine Crane, Colin Espie, Erika Forbes, Lucy Foulkes, Lorna Goddard, Allison Harvey, Erin Leichman, Lisa Meltzer, Jodi Mindell, Faith Orchard, Luci Wiggs and Michael Grandner. Thanks also to Fiona Ball, Sara and Matt Hunt and Robert Grieves as well as to Jenny Stock, Kitty Travers, Rebecca Mitchell, Rachel Jupp, Jim Martin, Ciara Bird, Sarah Aarons and Brian Sharpless. We are particularly grateful to the many families who took part in the pilot study; their responses and feedback have been enormously useful in helping us to develop the stories and sleep techniques in the book.

Alice would like to add personal thanks to her family, friends and colleagues. They are too numerous to mention all – but in particular, Paul (Wolf), Gerry and Joanna Gregory, Pat and Brian Heaps, Gerry Girou, Chris Bird, Lynne Wake, James Smithies, Rashad Braimah, Gabrielle Esu, Essi Viding, Thalia Eley, Mary Anderson-Ford, Maria Napolitano, Ana Richmond, Jason Ellis, Amber Gibbon, Chris French, Anna Gregory, Joe Shrapnel, Briony Weale, Ed Horrox, Terrie Moffitt and Avshalom Caspi. A particular thanks goes to next generation inspiration: her sons, Hector and Orson, nephews Holden and Harlan as well as Felix, Andre, William, Harry, Toby and Baby Alice.

Christy would like to add personal thanks to her family: Paul, Harry, Toby and Alice, as well as Julia and Roger Kirkpatrick, Amanda and Malcolm Wood, Mary and Michael Grigg, Mark Grigg and Mishka Diaz-Grigg and Sandra and Rory Burke. She would also like to thank other dear friends: Gemma Guyett, Nicola Parr, Vanessa Frances, Kim Bax, Ann Radford, Steve and Jo Pinches, Kath Jackson, Daryl Nilbert and Rachel Nasrallah. She is also grateful to her nieces and nephews: William, Eva, Daniel, Jemima and Zac, and is remembering and sending love to Lucy. Thanks also to Eva, Bede, Hector and Orson.

About the Authors

Alice Gregory

Professor Alice Gregory has been researching sleep for almost two decades and has published more than 100 scientific articles on sleep and associated topics. She completed her undergraduate studies at the University of Oxford in the UK, gaining a first class degree. After spending a year in Japan, Alice worked towards her PhD at the Institute of Psychiatry, London. She is currently a Professor of Psychology at Goldsmiths, University of London, UK. Alice is the author of the popular science book: *Nodding Off: The Science of Sleep from Cradle to Grave*. She contributes regularly to *BBC Science Focus* magazine and has also written pieces for *The Guardian, Balance* magazine and *GQ*. She has published articles with *The Conversation*, which have been republished in various outlets including *Sud Ouest* and *The Independent* and which have been read well over half a million times. She is happiest spending time with her family.

Christy Kirkpatrick

Christy Kirkpatrick is a freelance children's book writer. Christy obtained a first class degree from the University of Warwick, UK, before completing a master's degree in English (Modernism) from Royal Holloway, University of London in the UK. She went on to obtain a PhD in English, also from Royal Holloway. Her PhD explored writing and publishing in the early twentieth century. Christy spent a decade working in academic and educational publishing before becoming a writer. She has written books for children, teachers and parents for major publishers and has a particular interest in phonics and early literacy, sleep and special educational needs and disabilities. She lives with her husband and three children.

About the Illustrator

Eleanor Hardiman

Eleanor Hardiman is a Bristol-based illustrator and designer. Working mainly in watercolour, she creates serene pieces with a distinct and modern illustrative style. Eleanor also works frequently on editorial pieces, magazine covers and advertising projects over the world.

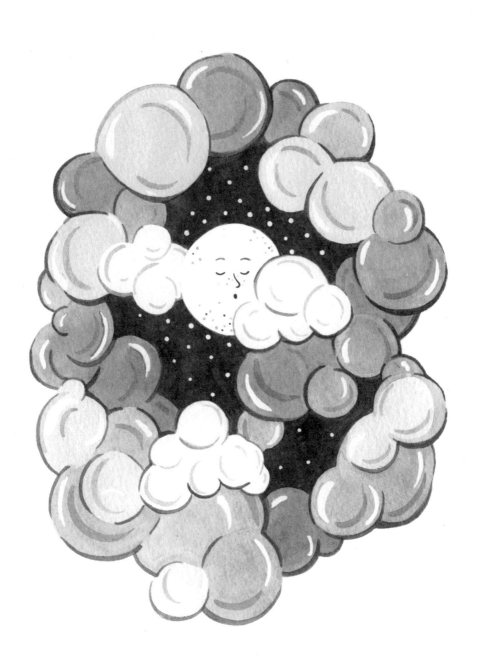

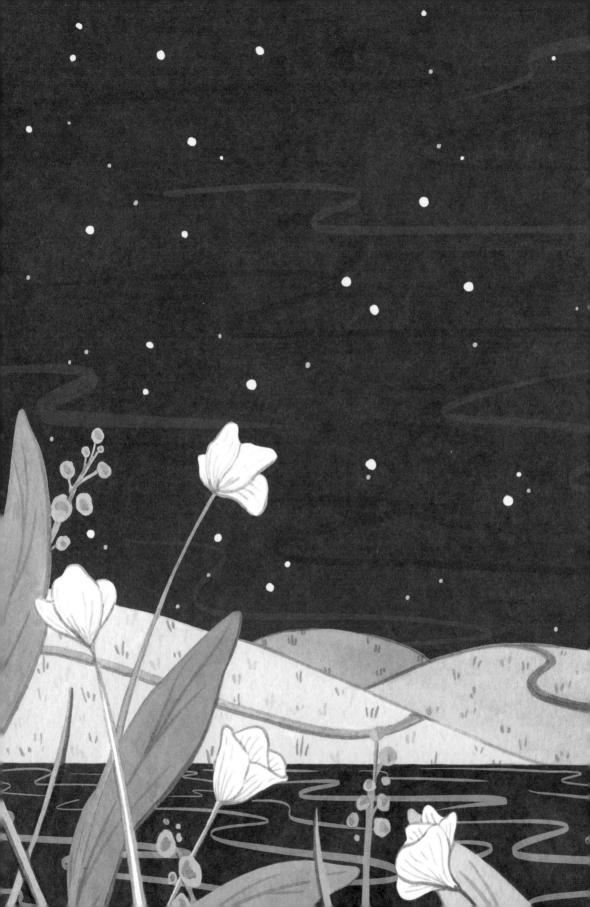